HIGH BLOOD PRESSURE

I0486031

202nm

Designed and written by:

Nester Kadzviti Murira

(c) N.K. Murira (2015)

This is a record of your health.

Carry this book wherever you go.

The information inside this book could save your life.

<u>Show this book to health personnel.</u>

Name:..

Address..

....

Tel..

In case of emergency contact:...

Tel...

Address..

Relationship...

Hospital/Dr...

Dr.'s Address..

....

....

....

....

My Current Medication is:

1...

2...

3...

4...

5...

6...

Allergies...

....

....

WHAT IS HIGH BLOOD PRESSURE?

The blood vessels narrow reducing the blood flow to the rest of the body and to the placenta, reducing blood flow to the unborn baby.

What causes High Blood Pressure?

It is not quite clear what causes this condition but there is some information that is known about it. It has been established that:

- A person who comes from a family in which one parent suffers from high blood pressure has a high likelihood to suffer from the condition.
- High blood pressure is also associated with high alcohol consumption and smoking.
- Extreme worry and stress
- High blood pressure is associated with excessive weight gain, a diet rich in fats and high levels of a substance called cholesterol in the blood.

How may a person with high blood pressure feel?

- One **feels breathless** on slight effort.
- One experiences **palpitations** or sudden fast beating of the heart as if one is frightened because the heart is under strain trying to push blood through the blood vessels that have toughened and narrowed.

- **The kidneys fail to function well**, there is reduced blood flow passing through the kidney and protein is lost through urine or one may have renal failure.
- **The brain is also affected**; one can experience severe headaches that do not respond to pain tablets. One of the small blood vessel may burst or rapture causing bleeding on the brain which causes stroke (mild or severe) depending on the size of the haemorrhage.
- **If one of the heart's small vessels bursts open, one can bleed into the heart muscle resulting in a heart attack.**
- Vision is affected and one may have blurred vision.

What are the signs of high blood pressure?

- One **feels extremely tired and breathless** on slight effort.
- Severe headache that do not respond to mild pain relief.
- **Swelling of feet and fingers**. The wedding or dressing rings become tight and dip into the fingers
- One may have **excessive weight gain** in mid-pregnancy.

What can one do?

The wisest action to take is to seek health advice immediately.

Follow the advice given by health personnel.

- Take the prescribed medication according to the advice given. Attend your review dates when expected and when you do not feel well.
- Eat fish, poultry (white meat) and vegetables proteins such as beans, peas, lentils.
- Eat lots of fruit and vegetables
- Reduce starchy foods and fatty foods.
- Reduce red meat like beef in your diet.
- Reduce intake of salt because it causes water retention in the body adding to the swelling.
- Avoid strenuous work.
- Make time to lie down and rest especially in the afternoons with feet elevated on a pillow.
- When seated, elevate feet on a stool to reduce swelling of legs.
- Take twenty to forty minute walks every day.

Have you taken your medication?

Please tick in the box

Date/Day	Morning	Afternoon	Evening	BP
Monday				
Tuesday				
Wednesday				
Thursday				
Friday				
Saturday				
Sunday				

Have you taken your medication?

Please tick in the box

Date/Day	Morning	Afternoon	Evening	BP
Monday				
Tuesday				
Wednesday				
Thursday				
Friday				
Saturday				
Sunday				

Have you taken your medication?

Please tick in the box

Date/Day	Morning	Afternoon	Evening	BP
Monday				
Tuesday				
Wednesday				
Thursday				
Friday				
Saturday				
Sunday				

Have you taken your medication?

Please tick in the box

Date/Day	Morning	Afternoon	Evening	BP
Monday				
Tuesday				
Wednesday				
Thursday				
Friday				
Saturday				
Sunday				

Have you taken your medication?

Please tick in the box

Date/Day	Morning	Afternoon	Evening	BP
Monday				
Tuesday				
Wednesday				
Thursday				
Friday				
Saturday				
Sunday				

Have you taken your medication?

Please tick in the box

Date/Day	Morning	Afternoon	Evening	BP
Monday				
Tuesday				
Wednesday				
Thursday				
Friday				
Saturday				
Sunday				

Have you taken your medication?

Please tick in the box

Date/Day	Morning	Afternoon	Evening	BP
Monday				
Tuesday				
Wednesday				
Thursday				
Friday				
Saturday				
Sunday				

Have you taken your medication?

Please tick in the box

Date/Day	Morning	Afternoon	Evening	BP
Monday				
Tuesday				
Wednesday				
Thursday				
Friday				
Saturday				
Sunday				

Have you taken your medication?

Please tick in the box

Date/Day	Morning	Afternoon	Evening	BP
Monday				
Tuesday				
Wednesday				
Thursday				
Friday				
Saturday				
Sunday				

Have you taken your medication?

Please tick in the box

Date/Day	Morning	Afternoon	Evening	BP
Monday				
Tuesday				
Wednesday				
Thursday				
Friday				
Saturday				
Sunday				

Have you taken your medication?

Please tick in the box

Date/Day	Morning	Afternoon	Evening	BP
Monday				
Tuesday				
Wednesday				
Thursday				
Friday				
Saturday				
Sunday				

Have you taken your medication?

Please tick in the box

Date/Day	Morning	Afternoon	Evening	BP
Monday				
Tuesday				
Wednesday				
Thursday				
Friday				
Saturday				
Sunday				

Have you taken your medication?

Please tick in the box

Date/Day	Morning	Afternoon	Evening	BP
Monday				
Tuesday				
Wednesday				
Thursday				
Friday				
Saturday				
Sunday				

Have you taken your medication?

Please tick in the box

Date/Day	Morning	Afternoon	Evening	BP
Monday				
Tuesday				
Wednesday				
Thursday				
Friday				
Saturday				
Sunday				

Have you taken your medication?

Please tick in the box

Date/Day	Morning	Afternoon	Evening	BP
Monday				
Tuesday				
Wednesday				
Thursday				
Friday				
Saturday				
Sunday				

Have you taken your medication?

Please tick in the box

Date/Day	Morning	Afternoon	Evening	BP
Monday				
Tuesday				
Wednesday				
Thursday				
Friday				
Saturday				
Sunday				

How does the disease affect the pregnancy?

It is now known that this condition affects first time mothers more than women who have had babies before. It occurs more in the rainy months

It is common in young women who lack family and spousal support.

It affects women who may have been hypertensive before pregnancy.

It affects pregnant women from mid pregnancy up to the postnatal period.

There is reduced blood flow to the placenta slowing down baby growth. The baby develops what is referred to as Intra Uterine Growth Retardation (**IUGR**). The baby is born weighing less than the expected weight (**Small for dates or small for gestation**) and looking smaller than is expected.

A pregnant woman with high blood pressure must:

- Listen to the baby's movements every morning and keep a record of how often the baby moves and take the record to the doctor or clinic when next she visits.
- Be prepared for a premature baby born by Caesarean section if the blood pressure remains high, to save both the mother and the baby's lives.

- If blood pressure continues to rise, the placenta suddenly separates from the mother's womb (**abruptio placenta**).

In abruption placenta,

- the mother feels sudden severe pain in the abdomen without any history of injury.
- Bleeding occurs and may flow out but sometimes it does not come out.
- The abdomen feels hard and pain persists. This is followed by fainting. This is an emergency! Both mother and baby are in danger! The baby may suffocate because of the bleeding and poor oxygen supply. The mother may collapse because of the bleeding.

Call the ambulance quickly or make arrangements to get to the hospital as soon as possible.

If the blood pressure continues to rise,

The pregnant mother may have convulsions (eclampsia)! This is an emergency!

One must get to the hospital as soon as possible. Both mother and baby are in danger! In both cases a Caesarean section is done to deliver the baby and control haemorrhage.

www.ingramcontent.com/pod-product-compliance
Lightning Source LLC
Chambersburg PA
CBHW072259200526
45168CB00016B/2190